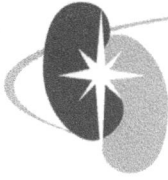

Renal Diet
Teaching You To Master Your He

I0071657

# Heart Healthy Living With Kidney Disease: Lowering Blood Pressure

## By Mathea Ford, RD/LD

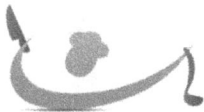

RENALDIET
HEADQUARTERS
BY HEALTHY DIET MENUS FOR YOU

# PURPOSE AND INTRODUCTION

What I have found through the emails and requests of my readers is that it is difficult to find information about a predialysis kidney diet that is actionable. I want you to know that is what I intend to provide in all my books.

I wrote this book with you in mind: the person with kidney problems who does not know where to start or can't seem to get the answers that you need from other sources. This book will provide information that is applicable to a predialysis kidney disease diet.

Who am I? I am a registered dietitian in the USA who has been working with kidney patients for my entire 15 + years of experience. Find all my books on Amazon on my author page: http://www.amazon.com/Mathea-Ford/e/B008E1E7IS/

My goals are simple – to give some answers and to create an understanding of what is typical. In this series of 12 books, I will take you through the different parts of being a person with pre-dialysis kidney disease. It will not necessarily be what happens in your case, as everyone is an individual. I may simplify things in an effort to write them so that I feel you can learn the most from the information. This may mean that I don't say the exact things that your doctor would say. If you don't understand, please ask your doctor.

I want you to know, I am not a medical doctor and I am not aware of your particular condition. Information in this book is current as of publication, but may or may not have changed. This book is not meant to substitute for medical treatment for you, your friends, your caregivers, or your family members. You should not base treatment decisions solely on what is contained in this book. Develop your treatment plan with your doctors, nurses and the other medical professionals on your team. I recommend that you double-check any information with your medical team to verify if it applies to you.

In other words, I am not responsible for your medical care. I am providing this book for information and entertainment purposes, not medical diagnoses. Please consult with your doctor about any questions that you have about your particular case.

# TABLE OF CONTENTS

Purpose and Introduction ..................................................3

Table Of Contents ............................................................5

The 411 on Kidneys and Heart Health...........................7

    What is Heart Health?...............................................7

    One Thing You Can Do Today to Improve Heart Health ......8

What is Heart Disease?...................................................9

    Types of Heart Disease............................................9

    What Causes Heart Disease? .................................16

Blood Pressure and Why It's Important...................21

    What is Blood Pressure?........................................21

    How does Blood Pressure Work? ..........................21

    Why is Blood Pressure Important to Heart Health? ..........23

    What is Normal Blood Pressure?..........................30

10 Tips to Heart Health with Chronic Kidney Disease ..........37

    10 Tips to Heart Healthy Living...........................37

How to Reduce Your Risk of Heart Attack by 33%.................49

    Ideas for Lowering Blood Pressure......................49

    Kidney Failure and Stress ....................................52

The Fabulous Four: Four Steps (you can take today) Toward Heart Health ..............................................................53

Other Titles By Mathea Ford: ....................................57

# THE 411 ON KIDNEYS AND HEART HEALTH

If you think of your heart as the engine that keeps everything running, you have a good sense of how it works in your body.

In the same way an engine powers a car, your heart powers your body. When you have a healthy heart, you can avoid many diseases and health challenges. Let heart health go downhill and you can see health problems begin. We are focused on understanding how heart health is tied to kidney health and how everything works together to create overall health for you.

## WHAT IS HEART HEALTH?

It's about taking care of your body so your heart is healthy, strong and able to provide you with all of the things that keep your body running like it should.

When you have good heart health, you can avoid a number of problems from stroke to heart attack, not to mention things like high blood pressure and decreased blood flow throughout the body.

A number of factors play into the health of your heart. For example, how you handle stress is a huge piece of your heart health, and your diet also plays a large role. People who are physically active and who enjoy a healthy diet often benefit from better heart health than those people who are inactive and eat poorly.

Because heart disease is progressive, it's important that you do everything you can to keep your heart working like the strong engine it is. When you suffer from other diseases, such as chronic kidney disease, it's even more important that you work to keep your heart healthy and strong.

Your kidneys are responsible for flushing your body of excess sodium and for helping to regulate your blood pressure. If your kidneys aren't working properly, they can't do their job, which can cause an increase in blood pressure and more stress on the heart.

Because you suffer from chronic kidney disease, it's normal to focus your attention on keeping your kidneys working properly, but it's unwise to ignore other elements of your overall health.

Therefore, while you might want to avoid dialysis, ignoring your heart is a mistake. It's more common for people to die of heart disease than to reach a stage 5 kidney disease.

Consider the information in this guide a roadmap for how to take better care of your heart. With tips, suggestions and solid information, it is a primer on how to give your heart the attention it deserves so it – and your kidneys – can keep working well for you.

### ONE THING YOU CAN DO TODAY TO IMPROVE HEART HEALTH

One of the most important things you can do is educate yourself about blood pressure because it is the leading contributor to heart disease. If you keep your blood pressure under control, you are at much less risk of heart disease and heart-related problems and you'll ensure that your kidneys aren't overworked from complications of high blood pressure either.

# WHAT IS HEART DISEASE?

Heart disease can manifest itself as a number of conditions including heart attack, heart failure, arrhythmia, heart valve problems and stroke. If you don't take care of your heart, or you have conditions that create heart problems, you can develop heart disease.

While many of these things can be a result of poor lifestyle decisions, many people have genetic conditions or other health problems that can contribute to heart disease.

## TYPES OF HEART DISEASE

There are five primary types of heart disease, and each presents its own set of problems, challenges, and treatment options and requirements.

### *HEART ATTACK*

When a part of the heart is blocked by a blood clot and that blood clot decreases the blood supply to that area, part of the heart muscle can die. This condition of decreased blood flow can exist for some time, but since there are deposits on the arteries that lead to the heart muscle, oxygen flow is decreased and eventually, can be cut off altogether, causing a heart attack. More than 1 million heart attacks occur each year. While you can recover from a heart attack, it can take about eight weeks for the heart muscle to recover and usually the heart has a lessened ability to pump as strong as before.

If you notice these symptoms, you should go to the nearest emergency room right away. Getting care within the first hour, if possible, is the best way to reduce the damage from a heart attack.

## Symptoms of heart attack in men

The "classic" symptoms of heart attack are those that men usually experience. Women should look for different symptoms, which are detailed next.

Some symptoms men should look for include:

- Heaviness or pain in the arm, chest, or just below the breastbone.
- A feeling like heartburn that can include a feeling of fullness or a choking feeling.
- Discomfort that radiates from the throat, arm, jaw or back.
- Shortness of breath, extreme weakness or a feeling of extreme anxiety.
- Irregular or rapid heartbeat (a feeling of your heart beating out of your chest).
- Breaking out in a cold sweat unexpectedly

Symptoms won't come and go, but will stay for a period of time and sometimes worsen the longer you feel them.

## Symptoms of heart attack in women

Women won't generally experience the same symptoms of heart attack that men experience. In fact, until recently, heart attacks were truly silent killers of women because the symptoms were often overlooked and women didn't know they were having a heart attack.

Some symptoms women should look for include:

- Chest pain or unexplained anxiety, which can be anywhere in the chest and might feel like a fullness or squeezing.
- Pain in the arm, neck or jaw. This particular symptom is more common in women than men and pain in the

arm won't just be focused in the left arm and the pain won't necessarily be intense, as it is in men.

- Stomach pain. This pain can be mistaken for the flu, a stomach ulcer or heartburn. Some women describe this pain as having a feeling like an elephant is on their chest.
- Lightheadedness, nausea, or breathlessness. Often women will feel very short of breath without exerting themselves at all. This may or may not be combined with chest pain.
- Sweating. This sweating will feel like stress-related sweating and it will be a cold sweat.
- Fatigue. Extreme fatigue that makes simple efforts like walking to the bathroom difficult can be a symptom of heart attack.

*IMPORTANT TESTS THAT CAN HELP DIAGNOSE HEART DISEASE*

When you have blood work done, your doctor might order a C - reactive protein test and a test for homocysteine. C-reactive protein is found in the blood; when there is inflammation in the body, the level of C - reactive protein will increase. The test can give your doctor a clearer picture of your risk of heart attack. Homocysteine is another hormone in your blood that can be very irritating to your blood vessels and high levels have been shown to affect your heart attack risk.

When the test shows inflammation in the body, it might be showing your doctor that you have inflammation in your arteries, which can show an increased risk of heart attack. Both of these levels can be lowered by ensuring you are eating a diet with plenty of B-vitamin rich foods and fiber.

This test alone cannot tell your doctor if you are likely to have a heart attack; the C - reactive protein test can also be used to diagnose or show an increased risk for lupus, certain types of cancers and some kinds of arthritis.

## HEART FAILURE

Many of us get a little uneasy when we hear the term "heart failure" but it doesn't mean that the heart has stopped working. It does mean that the heart is no longer pumping as well as it should.

Heart failure (commonly also called "congestive heart failure") is one of the most common health conditions in the United States; it affects nearly 6 million Americans and nearly a half million new cases are diagnosed each year. In fact, it's the most common cause of hospitalization for people who are older than age 65.

There is no cure for heart failure, but there are treatment options which include diet, lifestyle changes, and treatment of underlying medical issues.

You are more likely to develop heart failure if you:

- Are older than 65
- Are African American
- Are overweight
- Have already had a heart attack
- Are a man

## ARRHYTHMIA

Arrhythmia is a fancy way of saying that something is wrong with the rhythm of the heartbeat. The heart might beat too quickly, or too slow, or it might beat with some kind of irregular rhythm. You might have heard the terms "tachycardia" and "bradycardia". Tachycardia means the heart beats too quickly, while bradycardia means the heart beats too slowly.

Many people have arrhythmias with no other problems and can live life normally, but some arrhythmias are very serious. During these arrhythmias, there might be a lack of blood flow throughout the body and this can cause damage to the heart, the brain or other organs.

Arrhythmia occurs because electrical signals that control the heartbeat are somehow not working correctly.

Some of the things that can cause arrhythmias include:

- Smoking
- A heart attack, high blood pressure, heart failure or thyroid problems
- Diabetes
- Sleep apnea

There are usually no symptoms when you have an arrhythmia, but there can be some symptoms sometimes. These might include:

- Heart palpitations (you might feel like your heart has skipped a beat or is beating too hard)
- An irregular heartbeat
- A heartbeat that's slow

Sometimes the arrhythmia is more serious and can cause symptoms that are more serious and should be brought to the attention of a doctor. These include:

- Anxiety
- Fainting or almost fainting
- Sweating
- Chest pain
- Shortness of breath

HEART VALVE PROBLEMS

When one of the valves of your heart doesn't work well, you have heart valve problems, or heart valve disease. The heart has four valves – the tricuspid, mitral, aortic and pulmonary. Each of these valves has tissues that repeatedly close and open with each beat of your heart. The flaps are responsible for ensuring that the blood flows in the right direction through your body and through the heart's four chambers.

Sometimes, a valve's flaps won't close tightly and blood can leak into the chambers rather than going where it should – to an artery or through the heart. For Americans with valve problems, the most common cause of this is prolapse, which is when the flaps bulge back or flop into an upper heart chamber when the heart beats. Some of the things that can play into whether or not you will have valve problems include congenital defects and heart disease.

If valve disease is not treated, it can lead to stroke, blood clots, heart failure and even death from sudden cardiac arrest.

There is no medication that can cure heart valve disease, but lifestyle changes are often successful in mitigating complications from the disease.

### STROKE

A stroke occurs when blood flow to the brain is somehow cut off or an artery that feeds the brain ruptures. Stroke is a condition that can cause long-standing problems so recognizing symptoms of a stroke and dealing with it quickly are essential components to recovery.

There are many risk factors for stroke, including:

- Being male and over age 55
- Family history of stroke
- Smoking

- Heavy alcohol use
- The use of birth control
- Diabetes
- Obesity
- High cholesterol and/or cardiovascular disease
- High blood pressure

If medical treatment is sought quickly, in most cases people can recover from a stroke fairly successfully. But it's important that you understand what a stroke looks like so you can identify it and deal with it quickly.

Some symptoms of stroke include:

- A sudden and very severe headache
- Double vision, blurred vision, or trouble seeing with 1 or both eyes
- Speech problems
- Confusion
- Trouble walking, dizziness, loss of balance and coordination
- Weakness, paralysis or numbness on one side of the body

Sometimes people will have a "mini stroke" or what's called a transient ischemic attack (TIA) before they have a full stroke. This will bring on symptoms similar to stroke, but they will be mild and will pass. But often this mini stroke will precede the full, or massive, stroke.

If you notice these symptoms, you should go to the nearest emergency room right away. Getting care within the first hour, if possible, is the best way to reduce the damage from a stroke.

## WHAT CAUSES HEART DISEASE?

We've talked briefly about some of the risk factors for the above conditions, but let's look more specifically at how some conditions can put you at a greater risk of heart disease.

### Blood pressure

Blood pressure that is uncontrolled over a long period of time can damage blood vessels and heart muscle. When blood pressure is high, it can damage the heart because the blood is at high pressure in the arteries at all times. When this pressure is high, the heart has to work harder to pump blood.

As the heart works hard, it becomes bigger and stiffens. The heart works hard to try and continue pumping blood, but eventually it gets weak and fails.

Ultimately the weakened heart makes you more at risk for heart attack, sudden cardiac death and heart failure.

### Diet

A poor diet can cause serious damage to your heart.

For example, when you eat too much cholesterol, saturated fat, or trans-fat in your food, you can increase the levels of cholesterol in your blood. This can lead to the hardening of the arteries as well as stroke and heart attack.

When you eat a diet that's high in sodium, you run the risk of increasing your blood pressure.

Even if you aren't prone to sprinkling salt on your food, you should always read food labels because sodium is hidden in nearly every food we eat. It's at extremely high levels in packaged foods, but you'd also be surprised how much sodium is in canned food too.

If you eat out often, you should also research favorite menu items to see how much sodium is in those foods; some of the worst high sodium culprits are found in restaurants.

## Hereditary causes

You'll likely know if there is a family history of heart problems. If there is, you are at a higher risk of having heart problems. It's also important to know that if your brother or father developed heart disease before age 55 or if a mother or sister developed it before age 65 because you are at an even greater risk of having heart problems.

There are other factors that can contribute to an increased risk of heart disease that you have no control over. These include:

- Your age (the older you get, the greater the risk of heart disease)
- Your race (you are at a greater risk if you are African American, Mexican American or American Indian)
- Your gender (Men have a higher risk of heart disease than women)

## Diabetes

People with diabetes are at a much greater risk of heart attack and stroke than people without diabetes. Studies have shown that people with diabetes can also develop heart disease at much younger ages than people without diabetes.

Are you middle aged and with type 2 diabetes? If so, your risk of heart attack is as high as someone who does not have diabetes and who has already had one heart attack.

If you have diabetes and other conditions, such as high blood pressure, obesity or high cholesterol, your risk of heart attack is even greater.

## Stress

We all experience stress. That's just a fact of life. But if you experience long periods of unrelieved stress, you could be at a higher risk of heart attack and other heart-related problems.

One condition that you could develop if you have chronic stress is called atherosclerosis, a condition in which plaque builds up in your arteries. When you are stressed you are more likely to have high blood pressure, high cholesterol and an inactive lifestyle. All of these are contributing factors to atherosclerosis, a disease that can be a precursor to coronary artery disease, peripheral artery disease, and stroke.

**Metabolic syndrome**
Having one component of metabolic syndrome means you're more likely to have others. And the more components you have, the greater are the risks to your health.

If you are diagnosed with metabolic syndrome, your doctor is simply saying that you have more than one of the following conditions:

- High blood pressure – over 130/85
- High blood sugar level (pre-diabetes or diabetes) – fasting blood sugar over 100 mg/dL
- Overweight (most relevant if you are "apple shaped" and carry most of your weight around your middle) – waist bigger than 40 inches for men or 35 inches for women
- High cholesterol levels – HDL (good) cholesterol less than 40 mg/dL in men or less than 50 mg/dL in women
- Triglyceride levels over 150 mg/dL

The more conditions you have, the greater your risk of developing heart disease.

There are some things that can increase your risk of developing metabolic syndrome. These include:

- Race – People of Hispanic and Asian origin are generally at greater risk of developing metabolic syndrome than people of other races.
- Age – The older you get, the greater your risk of developing metabolic syndrome. The condition affects fewer than 10 percent of people in their 20s, but as much as 40 percent of people in their 60s.
- Diabetes – If you have a family history of diabetes or you had gestational diabetes, you are at a greater risk of developing metabolic syndrome.
- Obesity – If you have a BMI (or body mass index) of greater than 25, your risk of developing metabolic syndrome greatly increases.
- Other disease – If you have high blood pressure, fatty liver disease, cardiovascular disease or polycystic ovary syndrome (or PCOS), you have a greater than average risk of developing metabolic syndrome.

Having metabolic syndrome increases your risk of developing heart disease because each of the conditions that play into metabolic syndrome is a challenge to your heart health.

If you think you might have metabolic syndrome or you have several conditions that indicate metabolic syndrome, talk to your doctor so he or she can assess your risk factors for this condition. You should exercise for at least 30 minutes per day (check with your doctor) and work to control your blood pressure and blood sugar levels to improve your health.

# Blood Pressure and Why It's Important

## What is Blood Pressure?

Blood pressure is a reading that shows how hard the heart is working to pump blood throughout your body. If there are conditions that make this process harder, you will have an elevated blood pressure reading. However, some people suffer from low blood pressure and that can also be a health concern.

## How does Blood Pressure Work?

Each time your heart beats, it is pumping blood throughout your body so that the muscles can get the oxygen they need. To send the blood throughout the body, the heart pushes your blood through arteries, which are a network of strong blood vessels.

When the blood is traveling through the arteries, it is pushing against the sides of the arteries and the strength of the pushing is referred to as blood pressure.

When the heart is squeezing and pushing the blood through arteries, your blood pressure naturally goes up and when the heart relaxes, the blood pressure goes down. Each heartbeat results in a maximum blood pressure and a minimum blood pressure.

When you see your blood pressure displayed as two numbers – say, 120/80 – you are seeing those maximum and minimum numbers. The top number is the highest that your blood pressure reaches when the heart is squeezing and is called your systolic blood pressure. The bottom number (or second number) is the lowest that your blood pressure reaches when your heart is relaxing or resting; it's called your diastolic pressure.

*HOW DO YOUR KIDNEYS CONTROL BLOOD PRESSURE?*
Your kidneys have the very important job of removing excess waste products from the blood. There are two specific ways that the kidneys can impact blood pressure.

- Electrolyte processing. It's natural for the body to want to keep the levels of sodium and other specific minerals found in the blood at a consistent concentration. When there's excess sodium in the blood, the kidneys get a message that they must get rid of sodium through urine. If the kidneys are damaged in some way and cannot remove the salt, the body will retain extra water as it tries to dilute the extra salt that's in the blood.
- When this happens, there is an increased amount of liquid in the blood, which increases it volume. This, naturally, increases blood pressure because of the increased blood volume pushing against the sides of the blood vessels in your body every time your heart pumps.
- Renin. The kidneys monitor the amount of blood flowing through the renal arteries and if blood flow drops for any reason, it will secrete renin, a hormone that increases blood pressure. This hormone can help increase blood pressure if it gets too low, but it can also lead to a dangerously high blood pressure if the blood flow to the kidney is decreased.

*HOW ARE GLOMERULI IN YOUR KIDNEYS AFFECTED BY BLOOD PRESSURE?*
If your heart is pumping hard to keep blood flowing through the body, it can affect many organs and processes. Your glomeruli are clusters of blood vessels that help to filter the

blood and waste products; if you have kidney disease, you have a decreased amount of glomeruli working in a capacity that can help to filter waste and keep body healthy. This happens over time, because the glomeruli are made up of capillaries (very small blood vessels) that can be damaged easily when the blood pressure is increased. Over time, they lose function and decrease your GFR.

The glomerular filtration rate (GFR) measures how well the kidneys are filtering waste from the blood. A person's GFR is estimated based on a routine measurement of creatinine in the blood. Creatinine is a waste product that develops as a natural process when muscle cells break down. Healthy kidneys will take the creatinine out of the blood and send it to the urine to leave the body, but when kidneys aren't working well, the creatinine can build up in the blood.

## WHY IS BLOOD PRESSURE IMPORTANT TO HEART HEALTH?

Because your blood pressure reflects how hard your heart is working, it's directly related to your heart's overall health level.

There are many risk factors for heart problems, most of which are lifestyle related and which can be controlled.

### WHAT AFFECTS BLOOD PRESSURE?

There are a number of factors that can affect your blood pressure. These include weight, stress, medications, the kidneys, diabetes, smoking, a poor diet and other health problems.

### Weight and BMI

Your weight and your BMI (body mass index) are major contributing factors to blood pressure and your overall heart health. When you're overweight, you're requiring your heart to pump harder to sustain you throughout the day to reach all your tissues. Your Body Mass Index is considered a fairly reliable indicator of overall fat levels, but some people have bones that are heavy or they are naturally heavier, which can give them a higher BMI. So while your BMI is important, don't use it as the only indicator of health. There are many things that can also paint a picture of overall health.

Your BMI is just a simple calculation of weight and height. To figure your BMI, you should first know how tall you are and how much you weigh. Once you have that information, you can plug it into a BMI calculator to get your BMI.

One reliable calculator is found at the National Institutes of Health website: http://www.nhlbi.nih.gov/guidelines/obesity/BMI/bmicalc.htm.

A person who is 5'6" and weighs 150 pounds will have a BMI of 24.2, which is considered normal.

- If you have a BMI under 18.5, you are classified as underweight.
- A BMI of 18.5-24.9 places you in the normal weight category.
- If you have a BMI of 25-29.9, you are considered overweight.
- If your BMI is over 30, you are classified as obese.

**Weight and waist/hip ratio**
Another indicator that health professionals use to determine you overall health and heart health is your weight to hip ratio.

The WHR, as it's called, helps to determine how at risk you are (if at all) for weight-related health issues, including heart problems. Research has generally shown that people who are "apple-shaped" (or who carry most of their weight around their waist) are more at risk for health problem than those who are "pear shaped" (or who carry more weight around their hips).

A WHR of more than .90 for males and .85 for women can put someone into a dangerous category for health problems.

Here is a good calculator for determining your WHR: http://www.amh.org/healthresources/wellness-tools/health-calculator/waist-to-hip-ratio/

When you measure your waist, measure it at the smallest point; if you have a larger belly and don't have a definable waist, measure your waist about one inch above the belly button. Measure the hips around the widest point.

Some believe that the WHR is a more accurate way to predict future health problems since it takes into account body structure, which BMI does not do. However, some studies have shown that the number of people worldwide who are classified as obese would triple if the WHR were used to classify obesity instead of BMI.

It is important to note, however, that people who are obese can have a healthy WHR but still need to lose weight in order to avoid health problems. Therefore, many health care professionals like to use both measurements so they can develop an accurate picture of a person's health risk based on weight.

**Salt intake**

If you read labels, you might be surprised at how much sodium is in the majority of foods we eat on a regular basis. While the recommendation is for 2,300 mg of sodium a day, most Americans get far more than that.

When sodium enters the bloodstream, it changes the electrolyte balance in the body; this causes fluids to leave the cells and they enter the bloodstream to restore the electrolyte balance. This increases the volume in the blood vessels and increases blood pressure. The salt also causes your body to retain water to dilute the concentration in the body's cells as well.

Eating too much sodium is also hard on the kidneys, because when sodium intake is high, the kidneys get a signal to remove more sodium from the body, which increases urine output. But this places more stress on the kidneys and over time, they simply can't keep up. As they slow down and become less effective, your blood pressure can rise. Damage to your kidneys also results from the increased blood pressure as well.

While eating a high-sodium meal now and then won't cause high blood pressure, long-term and regular intake of high sodium foods can cause chronic blood pressure problems, which lead to other health problems.

Sodium is hidden in many foods; while most of us know the risks of eating fast food and processed food due to their high sodium levels, you might not know that breakfast cereals, vegetable juices, deli meats, jarred spaghetti sauces, and nuts are also high in sodium. Reading labels and identifying serving sizes and amount of sodium per serving is very helpful to your quest to lower your salt intake.

## Smoking

If you smoke, you are no stranger to the news that it's bad for your health. The backlash against smoking is great these days, but that's for good reason. It's been reported that as much as 20 percent of all deaths from heart disease in the U.S. can be attributed to cigarette smoking. The primary reason for this is that smoking is a major cause of coronary artery disease (heart damage).

The nicotine in cigarettes is largely the problem. It decreases oxygen to the heart and increases blood clotting. It can damage the cells that line the coronary arteries (arteries on your heart) and increase heart rate. In general, nicotine narrows blood vessels and makes your heart work harder. All of these things can increase blood pressure.

## Stress

According to the American Heart Association, the solid link between heart disease and stress isn't quite clear, but some things are true. When you are stressed, you might make decisions that are ultimately bad for your heart. You might drink more alcohol or get too little sleep. You might eat poorly (thus increasing cholesterol levels and perhaps leading to weight gain) and you might not exercise.

Especially if you are very stressed for a period of time, your body might release adrenaline, which can cause your breathing and your heart rate to increase. These things can be part of what's called the "fight or flight" response; the increase in heart rate and breathing can lead to higher blood pressure. When your body goes through the cycle of "fight or flight" continually, it causes your blood pressure to remain high over a long period of time.

## High cholesterol

When you have too much cholesterol in your blood, the arteries become narrowed because the cholesterol builds up on the walls of the arteries. This narrows the arteries and makes it harder for the blood to carry oxygen to the heart; when very little oxygen and blood reach your heart, you can experience chest pain.

There are two primary forms of cholesterol – the "good" cholesterol (or HDL) and the "bad" cholesterol (or LDL). HDL can clear cholesterol from the blood while LDL is the main product that can clog arteries with plaque. Think about the LDL cholesterol like garbage that is brought into your body through cholesterol in food, saturated fat and trans fat. Think about HDL cholesterol like a garbage truck- increased mainly via exercise – and it's something that goes around and picks up the garbage in your body. You want more garbage trucks so they can take all the garbage back to your liver.

Levels that your cholesterol should be to reduce your risk of a heart attack or stroke:

- o Total Cholesterol less than 200 mg/dL
- o HDL (Good) Cholesterol should be 60 mg/dL or higher as a woman and 55 mg/dL or higher as a man
- o LDL (Bad) Cholesterol should be 100 mg/dL or lower
- o Triglycerides should be less than 150 mg/dL

**Medications and blood pressure**
Cold medications can be dangerous for people with high blood pressure because many of them contain an ingredient that raises blood pressure. Most over-the-counter cold remedies contain decongestants, which can raise blood pressure. The decongestants work by narrowing blood vessels in the nose, which helps to relieve nasal stuffiness; but this affect can also apply to other blood vessels in the body, which can raise blood pressure.

These are the decongestants you want to avoid if you have high blood pressure:

- o Pseudoephedrine
- o Ephedrine
- o Phenylephrine

- Naphazoline
- Oxymetazoline

There are a few cold medicines that are designed for people who have high blood pressure. One of the most common is Coricidin HBP, which does not contain decongestants. But it does contain other drugs that can be dangerous if taken in high doses, so follow the dosing instructions carefully.

Some medications given for conditions like ADHD can also raise blood pressure.

## Caffeine
If you are fond of caffeine products or energy drinks, you might also suffer from high blood pressure related to using these products since caffeine causes the heart rate to rise. In fact, people who already have high blood pressure have to carefully watch how much caffeine they consume, and stick to about 2 cups of coffee per day maximum, but it is best to eliminate it altogether if you can.

## Kidney problems
If you have chronic kidney disease or other kidney issues, you have to keep a careful eye on your blood pressure. The hard work they do to keep your blood pressure even and help keep the blood flowing properly can tax them.

The research shows that high blood pressure makes your kidneys fail faster – and that you can have high blood pressure and not even know it. Once you know that you have kidney failure, make sure you are taking the extra steps to continue to control blood pressure – or get your blood pressure under control. When you lower your blood pressure, you prolong the life of your kidneys.

**Diabetes**

When you have diabetes, you are at increased risk of high cholesterol, which narrows blood vessels. In turn, narrowed blood vessels can lead to hypertension. The narrowed blood vessels don't pump the usual and right amounts of blood through the body, which can cause the heart to work harder and increase blood pressure.

People with diabetes should keep an even closer eye on their blood pressure. In general, doctors of patients with diabetes like to see blood pressure readings of under 130/80, though lower readings are better.

## WHAT IS NORMAL BLOOD PRESSURE?

Normal depends on many things. While there are "normal" ranges that apply to most people, some people will have a different standard depending on their general health and the presence of any health conditions.

If you have chronic kidney disease, your ideal blood pressure is 130/80 or below.

In the past, doctors were more focused on the "bottom" number (or second number) because it indicates how much pressure is on the arteries even when the heart is at rest, but these days, doctors consider both numbers to be critically important.

### WHEN IS BLOOD PRESSURE A CONCERN?

Blood pressure is a concern when it's elevated over a period of time. Many of us (though not all) will find that our blood pressure is normally high when we visit the doctor or after certain activities. Maybe for you, taking your blood pressure right after eating is a bad idea; if you ate a meal high in sodium or drank a large cup of coffee, you might get a reading that's high but not indicative of your true and normal blood pressure.

Blood pressure is only a concern when it registers high (or low) on a regular basis. When it appears to be a chronic (and regular) problem, that's when doctors become concerned.

## WHAT ABOUT LOW BLOOD PRESSURE?

While you might look upon someone who has low blood pressure with some envy, there are legitimate concerns with blood pressure that is too low on a regular basis. Low blood pressure is blood pressure that registers 90/60; this reading or anything lower can be a real concern.

Most doctors believe that low blood pressure isn't a concern unless it causes symptoms. But if you are experiencing any of the following symptoms, your doctor might want to do some intervention.

- Dizziness
- Unusual thirst or dehydration
- Blurred vision
- Nausea
- Fatigue
- Depression
- Inability to concentrate
- Fainting

Many of these symptoms mimic those of high blood pressure, so if you have any of the following risk factors for low blood pressure, talk to your doctor. Some include:

- Taking prescription medications like beta blockers or diuretics
- Heart problems
- Endocrine problems like under-active thyroid and low blood sugar
- Prolonged bed rest

- Lack of B-12 or folic acid

*DANGERS OF HIGH BLOOD PRESSURE*
When you have high blood pressure, your heart is asked to work very hard to pump blood throughout the body, something that can tax it greatly. This can cause a number of health problems.

Some of the main concerns with high blood pressure include:

- Vision problems – Over time, high blood pressure can cause the blood vessels in the eye to bleed or burst. This can cause blurry vision or create other vision problems. In extreme cases, this can lead to blindness.
- Stroke – High blood pressure is one of the most common risk factors for stroke. It can cause a break in one of the weakened blood vessels in the brain, and blood can leak into the brain. Sometimes a blood clot will form in the brain which can block one of the narrowed arteries. In both cases, stroke can occur.
- Hardening of the arteries – This can lead to a host of health problems including heart disease and heart attack.
- Kidney problems – If you already have kidney problems, high blood pressure can greatly exacerbate those problems. If you don't have kidney problems, prolonged high blood pressure can create problems. When blood pressure is high, the kidneys have a hard time carrying on their important function.
- Sexual dysfunction – Men over the age of 50 run the risk of erectile dysfunction due mostly to their age, but men who have high blood pressure at a greater risk of ED because the limited blood flow can restrict blood flow to the penis and for some men this can cause problems with achieving and maintaining erections.

*MONITORING YOUR BLOOD PRESSURE AT HOME*
Probably one of the best things you can do for your overall health is monitoring your blood pressure at home. It's great to get the benefit of the very accurate machines at the doctor's office, but keeping a regular eye on your blood pressure is key, especially if you have health concerns or you have high blood pressure.

There are two ways to monitor your blood pressure at home: with a manual or digital monitor. You also have to consider cuff size, size of the machine and special features. Finally, if you don't have a monitor at home, you can always use store monitors.

## Manual monitors
Manual monitors aren't for everyone. They require a fair amount of coordination and dedicated focus. If you have any physical limitations such as vision or hearing problems or you can't do the hand movements necessary to inflate the bulb, this might not be the best option for you.

Many people like taking their blood pressure this way, though, because they know that there are no possible technology concerns and it keeps you in close touch with your blood pressure, because you can actually "hear" it. Manual monitors are also usually less expensive than digital monitors.  Make sure you sit quietly for at least 5 minutes prior to starting your measurement with your feet flat on the floor.

## Digital monitors
Digital monitors are great for a number of reasons. First, the machine does all the work for you. You don't have to trust yourself to hear the heartbeats right and you often don't have to inflate the bulb manually. Some digital monitors will record several days' worth of readings while others will print out

readings so you can take a record of your blood pressure to your doctor.

Most digital monitors will operate both by being plugged in and by battery, but be sure to check how your monitor will be powered so you get one that suits your specific needs.

If you don't get an accurate reading or you get an error reading, take your blood pressure again, but wait at least 10-15 minutes before making a second attempt. Be sure to take the cuff off and put it on completely again. Sometimes the error is due to incorrect positioning of the cuff.

## Cuff Size

It's important to use the right cuff size for your arm. If you use a cuff that's too small or large, you will either get continuous error readings or you will get a reading that's incorrect, perhaps much higher or much lower than your actual blood pressure. People with an upper arm circumference of more than 13" should use a large cuff.

You can buy blood pressure monitors that come with a large cuff if you need that, but most monitors will allow you to change out the cuff size so if one member of your family has a large arm, they can use the same machine as someone with a smaller arm. Simply change out the cuff when necessary.

## Store monitors

Store blood pressure monitors can be quite useful if you don't have a monitor at home and don't want to (or can't) buy one.

These monitors are easy to find in drugstores near the pharmacy. If you decide to use one, keep in mind that you will get the most accurate reading if you are resting for a few minutes before you take your blood pressure, so either sit down somewhere in the store for a few minutes, or sit at the blood pressure monitor for a few minutes before you slip your arm into the cuff with your feet flat on the floor.

# 10 Tips to Heart Health with Chronic Kidney Disease

If you want to have a healthy heart, you should eat right, exercise and make good lifestyle choices. These are all things you have likely heard before and that's for good reason – these things work.

The good news is you might already be doing some of these things on a regular basis. Others might not be hard to incorporate into your daily life. Before you know it, you'll be living a heart-healthy lifestyle with little effort (but great payoff!).

## 10 Tips to Heart Healthy Living

*EAT MORE FRUITS AND VEGETABLES.*
Yes, this is surely one you have heard before! But there's a good reason why doctors, nutritionists and dietitians implore you to eat more fruits and vegetables – they are good for you in more ways than you realize.

Fruits and vegetables offer no-fat, usually low-calorie and nutrient-dense ways to get your calories. They satisfy a sweet tooth, a need for crunch and fill you up because they are full of fiber. They are full of essential vitamins and minerals and can make your skin and hair look beautiful while fortifying your immune system.

These are all good things!

Your kidneys are responsible for regulating the amount of potassium in your body, so when your kidneys are unhealthy, it's a good idea to limit the amount of potassium you take in. Eat fruits and vegetables that are low in potassium to avoid problems.

Some examples of low potassium fruits include:

- Blueberries
- Grapes
- Pineapple
- Strawberries

Some examples of low potassium vegetables include:

- Lettuce
- Green beans
- Cauliflower
- Cucumber

Avoid fruits and vegetables that are very high in potassium. Some high potassium fruits and veggies include:

- Bananas
- Oranges
- Avocados
- Dried fruits
- Olives and pickles
- Pumpkins seeds
- Vegetable juice cocktail
- Baked potatoes

### CONTROL PORTION SIZES

Learning to control portion sizes can go a long way toward keeping you healthy and vibrant. When you eat too much at a sitting, you feel sluggish and tired after your meal. You also tax your system as it works extra hard processing and digesting all the food you ate.

When you exercise portion control, you will also likely take a step forward toward staying at healthy weight, which is of course, essential to a healthy heart.

Learn what a portion size looks like. You might be surprised to find that portion sizes for many foods are smaller than you think. For example, a portion of meat or chicken should be about the size of a deck of cards, while a portion of cheese is about the size of a pair of dice. "Choose My Plate", a USDA website, can help you with portion sizes.

## Mindful eating

Consider learning how to eat mindfully, which is a system of being thoughtful and completely in the moment when eating. When you eat mindfully, you focus on every sensation of your food as well as every bit of your surroundings. You take all of this in as a way to appreciate your food, focus on the food and slow down your eating so you have mindful intention when eating.

When you eat mindfully, you focus on the sights, smells and sounds of your food. You notice how the food looks on the plate (is it colorful or all one color?) and you notice what it smells like as it is put before you. You focus on the crunch of the peppers and carrots in your mouth and the interesting texture of the couscous or quinoa. Mindful eating is about more than just eating – it's about focusing on and appreciating all the elements of your meal. When you do this, you are less likely to overeat or eat mindlessly.

### EAT WHOLE GRAINS AND AVOID WHITE FOODS

You have likely heard this edict before, but it's always good to repeat this very useful tip – eat whole grains as much as possible and avoid "white foods".

Try this exercise: When you sit down to dinner tonight or tomorrow, take a close look at your plate. Ideally, it will be full of colorful foods, but if it's not, pay attention to the color of the foods. Do you have a roll on your plate? Is it white or brown? Is there rice? Is it white or brown?

Whenever you choose carbs, make sure they are brown carbs and not white carbs. That's a simplification of the "eat whole grains" edict, but it's an easy way to remember what your plate should look like.

These days, food manufacturers have made it easy to find whole grains; many foods – like pasta – are available in a whole grain version when previously the only version available was white.

## LIMIT "BAD" FATS

For optimum heart health, you should limit your consumption of "bad" fats, or those that can clog arteries and do nothing for your health.

You can't just cut fat from your diet altogether. Unsaturated fats like those found in nuts, fish and some oils like olive and canola are good for us in many ways. They can reduce your cholesterol and lower your risk of heart disease. They help to keep your skin healthy and your hair shiny. They are critically important to the smooth operation of your body systems.

All fats have the same amount of calories per tablespoon. Switching one fat for another does not save you calories or fat, but it can make a huge difference in the health benefits you derive from the food.

Saturated fats and trans fats are an example of "bad fats". The fats used in baked items and those used in fried items (which you should avoid as much as possible anyway) are usually examples of "bad" fats.  They are also found in red meat, full fat dairy products, eggs and the skin of poultry. Most fats that are liquid at room temperature (such as oils) are considered "good" fats; the more solid a fat is at room temperature, the more dangerous they are for you to eat.

You instead want to eat fats that are unsaturated or monounsaturated. Switch to canola, olive or grape seed oil. Eat fish to get essential Omega 3 fatty acids. Avoid full fat dairy products, but don't cut the fat entirely.

### CHOOSE HIGH-QUALITY (AND LOW FAT) SOURCES OF PROTEIN

Protein is important as it's an essential building block to keeping the body healthy. But you should always choose high-quality versions of those building blocks. Turkey is an amazing source of lean protein and fish is rich in fatty acids, but good for heart health.

If you must have a hamburger, choose a lean ground beef and eat just a simple burger with one patty; limit your hamburger eating to just once or twice a month. Focus the rest of the time on enjoying lean and high-quality sources of protein; and when you do eat meat, keep your portion to about 3 ounces and choose center cuts; avoid chuck roasts and fatty steaks.

If you haven't been a fish eater, try to learn to enjoy fish. It has so many great health benefits that it's a real detriment to your health to not eat fish.

If you like chicken, that's great, but fried chicken is not good. If you usually eat fried or sautéed chicken, learn to enjoy broiled, grilled or baked chicken. There are many excellent recipes for oven-fried chicken strips; if you're willing to try new techniques and new recipes, you might be surprised by the delicious results.

Don't forget about peanut butter. It provides a great non-animal source of protein, but is also high in fat, so use in moderation and save it for a special treat.

## REDUCE SODIUM CONSUMPTION

You likely know that a high-sodium diet can contribute to high blood pressure, so reducing sodium is an excellent way to reduce your blood pressure and therefore improve your overall heart health.

Having a high sodium diet also taxes your kidneys as they work harder to process that sodium and clear it out of the body. When you eat a lower sodium diet, you help your kidneys to do their hard work and do it as efficiently as possible.

You can substitute many delicious seasonings for salt, but avoid potassium chloride, which contains potassium and can be dangerous for people with kidney disease. There are a number of salt-free seasonings on the market these days and many of them impart a nice, savory taste to food without adding sodium.

You can use no-salt seasonings like Mrs. Dash products or you can add herbs to your foods. Try a squeeze of lemon over your fish or chicken, for example, or make a garnish of tomatoes and cucumber for your chicken.

## PLAN MEALS

If you have never taken the time to plan your meals, you might not understand the benefit in doing so. Planning meals is one of the best things you can do for your health.

When you don't plan meals, you are really at the mercy of your hunger. If you are very hungry and you haven't planned or prepped, you're more likely to take advantage of fast food or take-out options, neither of which will help you build and maintain a healthy heart.

Planning meals does take a little time, but the more you do it, the easier it becomes. Here are some tips:

Pick a day when you will grocery shop each week (for most people, this is Saturday or Sunday) and sit down to do your planning the day before.

Think about what is going on in the next week and plan meals accordingly. For example, if you have a late meeting one night, plan for a super simple meal or leftovers.

Write down a dinner meal idea for each day of the week; use family favorite recipes or mix things up a bit by finding healthy recipes you might like to try.

Write down the ingredients you need for each meal and then check your pantry, refrigerator and freezer for things you might already have and cross those off the list.

Now, do the same for lunches and breakfasts, but be willing for the sake of time and budget to eat the same thing more than once for breakfast and lunch; it's easier on the budget and on your time.

Once you have your list, do your shopping for the week.

Once you have your groceries home, do any advance prep work that you can do to make mealtime go faster. You might chop up vegetables or even brown ground turkey and store it in the fridge. You could wash your salad greens and put chicken in a marinade. Doing these things will ensure that you save time when making dinner, making it less likely that you'll succumb to the drive through.

*EXERCISE REGULARLY*

Exercise is the most natural wonder drug available. When you exercise, you do many great things for your body and nearly all of those add up to improvement in heart health.

Remember, you can simply walk for as little as 20 minutes a day and derive benefit. Shoot for 30 minutes a day five days a week. You can start small and build up; let it become a habit. Choose a time of day that works for you so you will be able to include exercise on a regular basis. For many people, morning works best because they can get up and do their work out and know that it's done for the day. Taking a walk late in the evening works best for others.

The key is to discover what will work best for you; when you do that, you nearly guarantee success.

Here are some benefits of exercise.

- It strengthens your heart and improves your cardiovascular system
- It helps your body use oxygen better by improving your overall circulation
- If you have heart failure, it can improve symptoms
- It increases your energy so you have the energy to do other things that are good for your health
- It lowers blood pressure
- It helps you reach a healthy weight, which improves heart health
- It helps to fight depression and reduce anxiety and stress
- It improves your sleep and helps you feel relaxed

*ASK ABOUT MEDICATIONS TO IMPROVE YOUR KIDNEY DISEASE*

If you have high cholesterol, ask your doctor about whether or not you should or can be taking a statin; this can lower cholesterol levels and help slow the progression of chronic kidney disease. The statins help kidneys by reducing kidney inflammation and can improve the function of kidney tissues.

*TAKE YOUR MEDICATIONS AS PRESCRIBED*
Your medications can't do their important work if you don't take them properly. It's important that you understand the medications you are on, what they can do for you and how to properly take them. Then follow the instructions for dosing.

If you have any questions about your medications, it's important that you talk to your doctor and inform yourself so you can do the best for your health.

## Daily Menus
Before we get a glimpse of a "good" meal day, let's look at a "bad" meal day, which typifies the diet of many Americans, unfortunately.

*For breakfast*

Many Americans eat nothing for breakfast (which is terrible for your health) or they grab a quick breakfast. This might include sugary cereal or white bread toasted with butter.

*For lunch*

While packing your own lunch is a frugal and healthy idea, most of us simply don't take the time or care to do this.

Instead, most people enjoy a fast food, deli or restaurant lunch. Even if you choose salad, your meal is likely dripping in sodium, calories and fat.

*For dinner*

Many Americans choose quick foods at home, like frozen pizza or hamburgers. If they take a little more time, they might end up with a marginally healthy dinner like baked chicken, baked potato and steamed veggies. If they are running to a child's baseball or ballet practice, dinner might be tacos from a fast food restaurant or something equally non-nourishing.

While this menu plan is fast and fulfills the need for quick food while on the go, eating like this isn't the only option when you are busy (or just tired). With a little advance prep (remember the meal planning we talked about?) you can create quick and healthy meals at home. Choosing to do this also saves a lot of money.

Here is an example of a "better" day.

*For breakfast*

High fiber cereal with nonfat milk is a great choice for healthy eating. Add a low-potassium fruit for an extra nutrient kick.

Not a cereal fan? Consider scrambled egg whites and vegetables. You can whip this up quickly when you have the vegetables already cleaned and cut in the fridge. Consider making egg "cupcakes" on Sunday – simply add meats and veggies to each of 12 muffin cups and then pour eggs you have whisked with some nonfat milk over the top. Bake in a 350 oven for about 12-15 minutes and pop these out when cool. Then reheat in the morning for a super-fast breakfast.

*For lunch*

Consider packing leftovers from dinner the night before or pack a quick salad; you can pack your salads a few days ahead and just grab one each morning. Don't forget to add a lean protein for your salad (such as tuna, chicken or even tofu) and some fruit to round out the meal.

*For dinner*

Season your salmon before you leave for work in the morning and bake it quickly when you get home, adding cut veggies to the pan to also cook. Whip up a quick salad for a great, easy side dish. Or make turkey chili and freeze in meal-size portions; simply pull one out the night before and heat it up for dinner.

If it's the right season, slice some strawberries for dessert.

# How to Reduce Your Risk of Heart Attack by 33%

You can reduce your risk of heart attack by 33% or more by simply reducing your blood pressure. It's not an insurmountable goal but one that will reward you in untold ways, but mostly with good health.

## Ideas for Lowering Blood Pressure

There are many things you can do to lower your blood pressure, but we're going to focus on three big things — exercise, eating right and reducing stress.

### *Exercise*

Learn to make exercise a habit and a priority and you will get the benefit of lowered blood pressure.

If going to the gym seems like a far off goal, start slow. If you have been very sedentary, start exercising by taking short walks around your yard. When you start to feel strong enough you can walk around the block. Slowly build on until walking not only brings you benefit physically, but you start to see it as a habit. You will begin to look forward to it because it will make you feel better and less stressed.

Yoga is an excellent, gentle exercise that reduces stress and lowers blood pressure. Even if you have never done stretching before or you feel tight, you can start yoga. Just do stretches and poses until you feel some discomfort and then stop. You will find that if you practice regularly, you'll be able to take the stretches further and further until you are fully doing them and enjoying every second. Other fitness regimes that can provide benefits similar to yoga include Tai Chi and pilates, both of which can help you to limber up while decreasing stress and reducing blood pressure.

*EAT RIGHT*

This means eating a diet low in sodium and high in fresh fruits and vegetables (low potassium versions of these, of course). Prep meals ahead if that works for you and avoid the drive through as much as possible. Avoid eating out in general and use your meal planning tips.

Don't assume that eating a healthy diet means lots of prep time in the kitchen. You can do a lot of the work ahead of time or even create shortcuts for favorite meals. Consider coming up with 10 really delicious but fabulously simple recipes for busy nights.

*REDUCE STRESS*

Stress is a major contributor to high blood pressure, so learning how to control stress is critically important. When you learn how to control stress, you also learn how to calm your body which reduces blood pressure. This one simple thing can change your life.

It might sound difficult, but it's worthwhile. NO matter what you face in life, you can learn to control stress. At the end of the day, it's really about this – you can't always control what happens to you in life, but you can control how you handle it.

**Tips for reducing stress**

Here are 12 simple ways to reduce stress, which leads to reduced blood pressure and improved kidney health:

1.  Exercise. It all keeps coming around to the same ideas, doesn't it? When you exercise, you calm yourself and naturally reduce stress. This helps to also reduce blood pressure.
2.  Journal. Put your thoughts and worries on paper. Some studies have shown that keeping a journal can greatly reduce stress. It sure can't hurt to try, right?

3. Meditate. It can be hard at first to learn to slow your breathing and focus on nothing other than your thought, but meditation is an excellent way to reduce stress.
4. Play games. Playing a game with a group of friends or family members can relax you and help you cope with all of life's worries.
5. Plant a garden. No joke! Studies have shown that people who garden have lower stress levels than people who don't. This is true even if you don't have a green thumb.
6. Listen to music and sing along. Doing this gives you an escape and a stress reliever. Let it all out and dance around. You'll be better for it.
7. Reduce your caffeine consumption. When you drink too much caffeine, you don't sleep as well, which can increase stress levels.
8. Make sure you get enough sleep on a regular basis. Only you know what your ideal number of hours is, but for most people, it's between 7 and 9 hours a night. Make a sincere effort to get your minimum ideal number of hours at least the majority of the time.
9. Have sex. Not with just anyone, of course. That might cause you stress! But if you are in a monogamous, committed relationship, having sex can be a great stress reducer.
10. Laugh. Watch a silly movie or head to a party full of easy-going friends. Laugh until your stomach hurts and experience the benefits that laughter brings.
11. Get out in nature. Some studies have shown that taking a hike or just driving through a forest or state or national park can have great stress relieving benefits.
12. Take a bath. Run some water, add some bubbles and get your favorite book. Giving yourself the gift of a

relaxing bath can do wonders for your outlook and response to stress.

## KIDNEY FAILURE AND STRESS

The health of your kidneys is directly related to your blood pressure. If you take steps to reduce your blood pressure, you will also benefit your kidneys, and you can slow the progression of kidney disease.

Stress causes that "fight or flight" response, which increases your blood pressure. Now that you know how to keep your stress down, make it a priority to help keep your kidneys healthy.

# The Fabulous Four: Four Steps (you can take today) Toward Heart Health

There are many things you can do to improve your heart health, as you have likely already learned. But if you want to get started immediately, there are four specific things you can do.

## Make a doctor's appointment

One of the first and most important things you can do for your heart health is go to the doctor and get a complete checkup. Some of the heart-related tests you should get or your doctor should order are:

- Blood tests -- Including c-reactive protein (which tests for inflammation in the body and can indicate the presence of heart problems), homocysteine (which helps your doctor determine your risk of heart disease) and LDL and cholesterol levels (which gives your doctor a picture of your potential for heart disease risk based on the amount of cholesterol in the blood).
- EKG or ECG -- An electrocardiogram is also often called an EKG or ECG and can show problems with the electrical activity of your heart. If you have a heart attack or doctors suspect a heart attack, they will order this test, but sometimes doctors will order it when you have not had any problems so they can get a baseline reading in case you have problems down the road. Each person's heart will give a unique report so it's sometimes helpful to have a baseline reading for your heart.
- Cardiac stress test -- The common ways for this to be administered are as a drug stress test or a treadmill

test. In short, doctors will induce stress to your heart in some way and then see how your heart responds. This can give your doctor a good picture of the overall health of your heart.

- Heart scan -- A heart scan is also called a coronary calcium scan and it provides pictures of your heart's arteries. Doctors look at the pictures to determine if there are calcium deposits in the arteries, which can clog arteries and possibly lead to heart attack. Heart scans can be a useful diagnostic tool for doctors to assess your heart attack risk before you have symptoms and when you have no other obvious heart attack risks. In general, most doctors will only order a heart scan if you have some risk factors for heart attack, such as smoking, family history of heart disease or high cholesterol or high blood pressure.

*EDUCATE YOURSELF*

Do just as you have been doing -- keep educating yourself! One of the best things you can do for your overall health is to educate yourself. Understand cholesterol and high blood pressure. Read health magazines and stay abreast of the current heart health research.

When you visit the doctor -- whether for a routine appointment or for heart tests -- ask questions until you really understand the answers. An educated patient is often a healthy patient.

*START WALKING*

And here it is again – the suggestion that you exercise! But it's here for a reason. When you exercise you can do so many great things for your heart from reducing stress and blood pressure to building your immune system and strengthening the muscle that is your heart.

Begin by doing only what is comfortable. As you feel stronger and healthier you can add time to your walking until you are walking 30 minutes (or between 1 ½ to 2 miles) a day. If you begin to feel even stronger, you can continue to add time until you are walking an hour a day. It might seem like a pipe dream now but with a little investment of time and sweat, you'll be there.

*KEEP A FOOD JOURNAL*
This might seem somewhat off topic, but it's not. If you are serious about adopting a heart-healthy lifestyle, you should pay close attention to what you eat and that should start now, with what you eat on a regular basis.

You might find that your diet is far from a heart-healthy one, or you might be surprised to find that you do some things right.

As you begin to change your diet to one that's rich in heart-healthy components, pay close attention to what you like to eat and what makes you feel good.

Keep the journaling simple; write down what you eat and when. Keep a separate sheet for each day of the week and then look over your notes periodically. You might find ideas for a meal you forgot that you loved and you might also want to congratulate yourself now and then when you see how much your diet has improved.

# OTHER TITLES BY MATHEA FORD:

**Mathea Ford, Author Page (all books):**

http://www.amazon.com/Mathea-Ford/e/B008E1E7IS/

The Kidney Friendly Diet Cookbook

http://www.amazon.com/Kidney-Friendly-Diet-Cookbook-PreDialysis-ebook/dp/B00BC7BGPI/

Create Your Own Kidney Diet Plan

http://www.amazon.com/Create-Your-Kidney-Diet-Plan-ebook/dp/B009PSN3R0/

Living with Chronic Kidney Disease - Pre-Dialysis

http://www.amazon.com/Living-Chronic-Kidney-Disease-Pre-Dialysis-ebook/dp/B008D8RSAQ/

Eating a Pre-Dialysis Kidney Diet - Calories, Carbohydrates, Fat & Protein, Secrets To Avoid Dialysis

http://www.amazon.com/Eating-Pre-Dialysis-Kidney-Diet-Carbohydrates-ebook/dp/B00DU2JCHM/

Eating a Pre-Dialysis Kidney Diet - Sodium, Potassium, Phosphorus and Fluids, A Kidney Disease Soluion

http://www.amazon.com/Eating-Pre-Dialysis-Kidney-Diet-Phosphorus-ebook/dp/B00E2U8VMS/

Eating Out On a Kidney Diet: Pre-dialysis and Diabetes: Ways To Enjoy Your Favorite Foods

http://www.amazon.com/Eating-Out-Kidney-Diet-Pre-dialysis/dp/0615928781/

Kidney Disease: Common Labs and Medical Terminology: The Patient's Perspective

http://www.amazon.com/Kidney-Disease-Terminology-Perspective-Pre-Dialysis/dp/0615931804/

Dialysis: Treatment Options for the Progression to End Stage Renal Disease

http://www.amazon.com/Dialysis-Treatment-Options-Progression-Disease/dp/0615932258/

Mindful Eating For A Pre-Dialysis Kidney Diet: Healthy Attitudes Toward Food and Life

http://www.amazon.com/Mindful-Eating-Pre-Dialysis-Kidney-Diet/dp/0615933475/